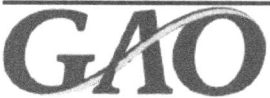

United States Government Accountability Office

Testimony

Before the Subcommittee on Early Childhood, Elementary, and Secondary Education, Committee on Education and the Workforce, House of Representatives

For Release on Delivery
Expected at 10:00 a.m. EDT
Thursday, June 27, 2013

SCHOOL LUNCH

Modifications Needed to Some of the New Nutrition Standards

I0428615

Statement of Kay E. Brown, Director
Education, Workforce, and Income Security

GAO-13-708T

GAO Highlights

Highlights of GAO-13-708T, a report to Subcommittee on Early Childhood, Elementary, and Secondary Education, Committee on Education and the Workforce, House of Representatives

SCHOOL LUNCH

Modifications Needed to Some of the New Nutrition Standards

Why GAO Did This Study

The National School Lunch Program served 31.6 million children in fiscal year 2012, in part through $11.6 billion in federal supports. The most recent reauthorization of the program, the Healthy, Hunger-Free Kids Act of 2010 required that nutrition standards for school lunches be updated. As a result, USDA issued final regulations aimed at providing lunches high in nutrients and low in calories that better meet the dietary needs of school children and required that they be implemented beginning in school year 2012-2013. The new rules provide detailed requirements for meal components—fruits, vegetables, grains, meats, and milk; update requirements for calories, sodium, and fats; and require that each student's lunch contain a fruit or vegetable. To provide information on challenges that school districts have faced, this testimony draws on work GAO conducted as part of its ongoing study of implementation of the changes. Specifically, GAO reviewed relevant federal laws, as well as USDA regulations, guidance, and studies; interviewed USDA officials and groups of food service officials and relevant industry representatives; and visited eight school districts. The districts varied by geographic location, size, and certain student and food services characteristics.

What GAO Recommends

GAO recommends that USDA permanently remove the meat and grain maximum requirements and allow flexibility to help districts comply with the lack of overlap in the calorie ranges for grades 6-8 and 9-12 lunches. USDA generally agreed with GAO's recommendations.

View GAO-13-708T. For more information, contact Kay E. Brown at (202) 512-7215 or brownke@gao.gov

What GAO Found

School districts faced several challenges implementing the new lunch requirements in school year 2012-2013, according to the eight districts GAO visited and food service and industry officials GAO interviewed from across the country; and the U.S. Department of Agriculture's (USDA) response to some of these challenges has been limited. For example, because USDA regulations restrict the amounts of meats and grains that can be served in school lunches each week, all eight districts GAO visited needed to modify or eliminate popular menu items. These changes sometimes led to negative student reactions. The meat and grain restrictions also led to smaller lunch entrees, making it difficult for some schools to meet minimum calorie requirements for lunches without adding items, such as gelatin, that generally do not improve the nutritional quality of lunches. In response to feedback from states and districts regarding operational challenges caused by the meat and grain restrictions, USDA lifted the limits temporarily, first for the remainder of school year 2012-2013 and then for school year 2013-2014. USDA officials said they did not see a problem making the temporary changes to help with implementation because the limits on meats and grains and the limits on the calories in lunches are somewhat redundant, as both address portion size. However, because the change was seen as temporary, the eight districts GAO visited made only marginal changes to their menus. Rather, several district food services officials, as well as relevant industry representatives, indicated the need for a permanent federal decision on these restrictions, which USDA has also acknowledged.

The calorie range requirements for lunches also challenged some districts, particularly those with schools that include students from both grades 6-8 and 9-12. Because the required lunch calorie ranges for these two grade groups do not overlap, districts with such schools face difficulties planning menus and serving lunches that comply with both requirements. For example, one food services official, whose district includes schools serving 7th through 12th graders, developed menus with calorie counts between the grades 6-8 maximum and the grades 9-12 minimum, leaving the lunches out of compliance with both sets of restrictions. Although USDA has acknowledged that menu planning in such schools can be challenging, USDA's current guidance does not provide these districts flexibility to assist their efforts to comply. Rather, guidance suggests that students from different grades be provided with different lunches, a solution that may be impractical in schools in which students of different grades share lunch periods and serving lines.

Although the eight districts GAO visited expressed support for the improvements to the nutritional quality of school lunch, they reported additional challenges meeting the new requirements, such as student acceptance, food waste, costs, and participation. For example, USDA requires that meals include whole grain-rich products and certain vegetables, but most districts noted that obtaining student acceptance of foods like whole grain pasta and beans has been challenging. If students do not accept these items, the result may be increased food waste or decreased participation in the lunch program, which were concerns in most districts GAO visited. However, student acceptance of the changes will likely improve over time, as indicated by their positive comments about healthy food and consumption of fruits and vegetables in most districts GAO visited.

_____ United States Government Accountability Office

GAO U.S. GOVERNMENT ACCOUNTABILITY OFFICE

441 G St. N.W.
Washington, DC 20548

Chairman Rokita and Members of the Subcommittee,

I am pleased to participate in today's discussion of school districts' experiences implementing the new requirements for the National School Lunch Program. This program served 31.6 million children in fiscal year 2012, supported in part through federal subsidies and commodities totaling $11.6 billion. Although federal requirements for the content of school lunches have existed since the program's creation, the Healthy, Hunger-Free Kids Act of 2010—the law that most recently reauthorized school meal programs—required that they be updated by the U.S. Department of Agriculture (USDA), which administers the National School Lunch Program. In response, USDA updated requirements for the content of lunches based on the recommendations of the Institute of Medicine.[1] USDA issued final regulations defining these new requirements in January 2012, and required the implementation of many of these requirements beginning in school year 2012-2013. USDA's updated regulations aim to provide lunches high in nutrients and low in calories that better meet the dietary needs of school children and protect their health. To that end, the regulations make several changes and additions to the previous requirements for the content of school lunches, such as the new requirement that each student's lunch contain at least one fruit or vegetable. Under agreements with state agencies, local school food authorities (SFAs), which are generally aligned with school districts, serve meals to children in schools and are the entities responsible for implementing these requirements.

As school year 2012-2013 has progressed, both USDA and the media have reported that states, SFAs, school officials, parents, and students have expressed some concerns about the school lunch changes. While the changes to school lunch are the primary school food changes required to be implemented in school year 2012-2013, the Healthy, Hunger-Free Kids Act of 2010 also required similar updates to nutrition standards for the School Breakfast Program and other foods sold in schools—or competitive foods—which will be implemented in future

---

[1] Pub. L. No. 111-296 § 201, 124 Stat. 3183, 3214. As required by the law, USDA updated the nutrition standards based on recommendations issued by the Food and Nutrition Board of the National Research Council of the National Academies of Science, part of the Institute of Medicine. Throughout this report, we refer to these as the Institute of Medicine's recommendations.

GAO-13-708T

school years. As a result, issues that have arisen because of implementation of the school lunch changes may have implications for future changes.

My remarks today will generally address challenges that school districts faced implementing the new school lunch requirements in school year 2012-2013. This information was gathered using several methods, including reviews of relevant federal laws, regulations, and guidance; interviews of USDA officials, a group of eight SFA directors representing both their own districts and their regions of the country, and a group of eleven relevant industry representatives;[2] and site visits conducted to eight school districts across the country. This work was conducted as part of our current study of implementation of the school lunch changes, in which we are assessing the extent to which school lunch participation changed during school year 2012-2013, implementation challenges, and USDA's assistance with implementation of the new requirements.[3] Our site visits were conducted between March and May 2013, and my remarks represent some of our findings from these visits. The school districts selected for these visits provide variation across geographic location, district size, and certain characteristics of the student population and district food services.[4] For example, we visited districts that generally prepare school lunches in one central kitchen before delivering them to schools, districts that prepare lunches in kitchens on-site in each school, and others that use alternative approaches for lunch preparation. Seven of the school districts we visited manage their own food service operations, while one district contracts with food service management companies. In each district, we met with SFA staff at the district and

---

[2] The School Nutrition Association (SNA), a national non-profit organization representing 55,000 members involved in serving meals to children in schools, assisted our efforts to speak with these groups. The eight SFA directors we spoke with were representatives on SNA's public policy and legislation committee, which includes representatives from each region of the country, as well as SNA's board of directors. None of these SFA directors were responsible for administering the National School Lunch Program in districts that we selected for site visits, and only one of the SFA directors was from a state in which we conducted a site visit. The 11 industry representatives we spoke with were members of SNA, and some serve on the Association's industry advisory board.

[3] We anticipate issuing a final report on this study in late 2013.

[4] We conducted site visits to Caddo Parish Public Schools (LA), Carlisle Area School District (PA), Chicago Public Schools (IL), Coeur d'Alene School District (ID), Fairfax County Public Schools (VA), Irving Independent School District (TX), Mukwonago Area School District (WI), and Spokane Public Schools (WA).

school levels, school administrators, and students, and we observed lunch in at least two schools of different grade levels. We also interviewed the eight state child nutrition program directors overseeing these districts. Although both public and non-profit private elementary and secondary schools, as well as residential child care institutions, participate in the National School Lunch Program, all of the districts we visited were public. We cannot generalize our findings from the site visits beyond the school districts we visited.

My remarks also reflect our reviews of relevant USDA data and studies. For example, we reviewed USDA's School Nutrition Dietary Assessment Study IV (2012), which provides information on school lunches and other foods sold in schools nationwide in school year 2009-2010.[5] Further, because it is the basis for USDA's revised regulations on the content of school lunches, we reviewed the Institute of Medicine's report, School Meals: Building Blocks for Healthy Children (2010).[6] We assessed the methodologies and findings of the studies we reviewed and determined that they were sufficiently reliable for the purposes of this testimony.

We conducted this work as part of our ongoing performance audit on implementation of the new school lunch requirements from February 2013 through June 2013 in accordance with generally accepted government auditing standards. Those standards require that we plan and perform the audit to obtain sufficient, appropriate evidence to provide a reasonable basis for our findings and conclusions based on our audit objectives. We believe that the evidence obtained provides a reasonable basis for our findings and conclusions based on our audit objectives.

Background

The National School Lunch Program, established in 1946, is intended to safeguard the health and well-being of the nation's children. The program provides nutritionally balanced low-cost or free lunches in participating schools to about 31 million children each month. At the federal level, USDA's Food and Nutrition Service oversees the program, which is

---

[5] U.S. Department of Agriculture, Food and Nutrition Service, Office of Research and Analysis, School Nutrition Dietary Assessment Study IV (Alexandria, VA: November 2012).

[6] Institute of Medicine, School Meals: Building Blocks for Healthy Children (Washington, D.C.: The National Academies Press, 2010).

administered by states and local SFAs. In fiscal year 2012, the federal government spent over $11 billion on the National School Lunch Program. Specifically, USDA provides reimbursement in the form of cash subsidies and donated commodities based on the number of lunches served that meet certain federal requirements. Although federal requirements for the content of school lunches have existed since the program's inception, as research has documented changes in the diets of Americans and the increasing incidence of overweight and obesity in the U.S., federal lunch requirements have become increasingly focused on improving the nutritional content of lunches.

The Healthy, Hunger-Free Kids Act of 2010, which most recently reauthorized the National School Lunch Program, required changes to the federal lunch requirements with the intention of reducing childhood obesity and improving children's diets. Since 1994, federal law has required SFAs to serve school lunches that are consistent with the Dietary Guidelines for Americans,[7] and in 2004, federal law required USDA to issue federal rules providing SFAs with specific recommendations for lunches consistent with the most recently published version of the Guidelines. As a result of that requirement, USDA asked the Institute of Medicine to review the food and nutritional needs of school-aged children in the United States using the 2005 Dietary Guidelines for Americans and provide recommended revisions to meal requirements for the National School Lunch Program. The Institute published its final report in 2010, and also in that year, the Healthy, Hunger-Free Kids Act of 2010 required USDA to update the lunch requirements based on these recommendations. The Institute's report recommended changes to the lunch component and nutrition requirements in place at the time. Regarding the lunch components—fruits, vegetables, grains, meats, and milk—the Institute recommended offering both fruits and vegetables daily, increasing whole grain-rich foods, offering only fat-free and low-fat milk, and limiting the amount of grains and meats/meat alternates served each week. Regarding the nutrition requirements, the Institute recommended including both minimum and maximum calorie levels for lunches, increasing the emphasis on limiting saturated fat and minimizing trans fat, and reducing

---

[7] The Dietary Guidelines for Americans were first issued in 1980, and most recently issued in 2010. The Secretaries of Agriculture and Health and Human Services are required, at least every 5 years, to publish a report entitled "Dietary Guidelines for Americans" based on current scientific and medical knowledge.

sodium content. USDA issued a proposed rule on the new lunch requirements in January 2011[8] and a final rule in January 2012.[9] The final rule required implementation of many of the new lunch requirements beginning in school year 2012-2013. Since the final rule was issued, USDA has provided extensive guidance, as well as technical assistance and training, to states and SFAs to assist with implementation of the new requirements.

The Eight SFAs We Visited Faced Several Challenges Implementing the New Lunch Requirements

All Were Challenged by Meat and Grain Limits

Because regulations issued in January 2012 by USDA placed limits on the amounts of meats/meat alternates and grains that can be included in a school lunch, all eight SFAs we visited modified or eliminated some popular menu items, leading to negative student reactions in some districts. USDA's new regulations specify the minimum and maximum weekly number of ounces of meats. cheese, or other meat alternates and the minimum and maximum weekly number of ounces of grains to be served with lunch, which differ by grade level.[10] In comparison, the previous regulations only specified the minimum number of ounces of meats and grains required to be served with lunch each week. (See table 1.) Officials in one of the districts we visited told us that, in response to the new limits, cheeseburgers were removed from the elementary and

[8] Nutrition Standards in the National School Lunch and School Breakfast Programs, 76 Fed. Reg. 2494 (proposed Jan.13, 2011) (to be codified at 7 C.F.R. pts. 210 and 220).

[9] Nutrition Standards in the National School Lunch and School Breakfast Programs, 77 Fed. Reg. 4088 (Jan. 26, 2012) (codified at 7 C.F.R. pts. 210 and 220).

[10] The new regulations also specify the minimum number of ounces of meats and grains that must be served each day but do not specify the maximum number of ounces of meats and grains that must be served each day.

middle school lunch menus because adding cheese to the district's burger patties would have made it difficult to stay within the weekly meat maximums. In another district, the SFA reported that it switched from using shredded cheese on the chili dog to processed cheese sauce because it does not count as a meat alternate. A similar type of switch occurred in one of the districts we visited because of the grain maximums. That SFA reported that it changed from serving a whole grain chip to a potato chip because the potato chip did not count as a grain. The grain maximums also affected popular lunch items, such as sandwiches. For example, four districts we visited reduced certain grain options used for sandwiches, such as the sub roll and the tortilla wrap, and two districts stopped serving peanut butter and jelly sandwiches as a daily option in elementary schools because the weekly grain maximum did not allow for a sandwich to be served every day. SFAs in four of the districts we visited noted that student reactions to these menu item changes were generally negative, and some said the changes had impacts on participation, that is, the number of students purchasing school lunches. For example, the tortilla wrap size change in one district was followed by a significant decrease in the number of students selecting their lunches from the previously popular deli sandwich line in the high schools, as well as a decrease in the overall percentage of students purchasing school lunches in those schools. Another district's change to its sub roll contributed to a middle and high school student boycott of school lunch that lasted for 3 weeks.

Table 1: The Previous Federal Requirements for Weekly Meat and Grain Portions in School Lunches Compared to School Year 2012-2013 Requirements

Grade Levels	Previous Federal Requirements - Minimums			School Year 2012-2013 Requirements – Minimums and Maximums		
	K-3	4-12	7-12[a]	K-5	6-8	9-12
Meat (in ounces)	7.5	10	10 or 15[b]	8-10	9-10	10-12
Grain (in ounces)	8 or 10[b]	8 or 12[b]	8 or 15[b]	8-9	8-10	10-12

Source: USDA Analysis of Previous and Current Requirements, 77 Fed. Reg. 4088, 4113.

[a]This was an optional grade configuration allowed under the previous federal requirements.

[b]Under the previous federal requirements for school lunch, SFAs could choose to use one of five approved approaches to plan their menus. Three of these approaches focused on nutrient requirements and did not specify portion size requirements. The two approaches that included portion sizes requirements differed in the minimum requirements for certain grade levels, as shown in the table.

To comply with both the meat and grain maximums and the required calorie minimums for lunches, some districts added foods that generally did not improve the nutritional value of lunches. In the new requirements,

USDA specified daily minimum and maximum calorie levels for school lunches by grade group (K-5, 6-8, and 9-12), which lunch menus must meet on average over the school week. However, because the entrée, typically consisting of meat and grain, generally provides the majority of the calories in the meal, the weekly meat and grain maximums that limit the size of entrées in effect also limited the calories of the lunches. As a result, five SFAs we visited reported that the meat and grain maximums made it difficult to plan menus that met the minimum calorie requirement for grade 9-12 lunches—750 calories. To comply, some SFAs added foods to the menus that, while allowable, generally do not improve the nutritional value of lunches. For example, in three of the districts we visited, the SFAs reported adding pudding to certain high school menus to bring the menus into compliance with the calorie minimum. Some SFAs also added gelatin, ice cream, or condiments such as butter, jelly, ranch dressing, or cheese sauce to become compliant, according to the districts we visited and the SFA and industry groups we spoke with. While these additional menu items provided needed calories to lunches, they also likely increased the amount of sugar, sodium, or fat in the meal, potentially undercutting the federal law's goal of improving the nutritional quality of lunches.[11]

Some SFAs noted that obtaining meat and grain products from food vendors that complied with the new requirements was a continual and evolving process during school year 2012-2013 because vendors were continually modifying products throughout the year. For example, four SFAs we visited said they met regularly with vendors during school year 2012-2013 as vendors worked to bring their products into compliance. One of those SFAs reported working closely with food manufacturers and vendors throughout the summer of 2012 to find appropriate products, including a 1.5 ounce burger patty—which is less than half the size of a ¼ pound burger—that allowed the district to continue to serve cheeseburgers to all students. Representatives from a group of food manufacturers and other relevant industries we spoke with indicated that the meat and grain maximums were challenging to respond to in part because the grain maximums had unexpectedly changed between the proposed and final rules, and the time between issuance of the final

---

[11]However, lunches in which these menu items are added must still comply with the new nutrition requirements, which currently include limits on the amount of fat in school lunches. Beginning in school year 2014-2015, the new nutrition requirements also limit the amount of sodium in lunches.

regulations and required implementation was short.[12] Some noted that while they were eventually able to reformulate their products to comply with the new requirements, the process took longer than the 6 months available between issuance of the final rule and the required implementation date.[13]

In response to feedback from states and SFAs regarding operational challenges caused by the meat and grain maximums, USDA lifted the maximums temporarily. First, in December 2012, USDA issued guidance allowing states to consider SFAs to be in compliance with the requirements for school year 2012-2013 if their menus exceeded the weekly meat and grain maximums. A few months later, in February 2013, USDA provided the same flexibility for school year 2013-2014, acknowledging that SFAs needed guidance to help with meal planning and food procurement for the coming school year, as SFAs often plan menus and order or contract for food beginning in the winter of the previous school year. The February guidance also stated that USDA understands the need for longer term guidance on this issue and is considering options for addressing the meat and grain maximums beyond school year 2013-2014. In May 2013, USDA officials told us that the Department wanted to be responsive to the challenges they had heard about, and they did not see a problem making the temporary change to help with implementation because the meat and grain maximums and the calorie maximums both accomplish the goal of addressing portion size,

[12] The weekly grain maximums for grades K-5 and 9-12 were higher in the proposed rule than in the final rule, as they changed from 10 to 9 ounces and 13 to 12 ounces, respectively. USDA officials explained that they made the change because they could not implement the proposed rule's limit on starchy vegetables due to a provision in the Consolidated and Further Continuing Appropriations Act of 2012, Pub. L. No. 112-55, which prevented USDA from implementing any maximum limits on vegetables. USDA officials said that they lowered the maximum weekly ounces of grains to limit the overall starchy items served with lunch. Concerning timing, the final rule was issued January 26, 2012 with implementation required by July 1, 2012, which was the beginning of school year 2012-2013.

[13] Some industry representatives noted that because of the need to focus on product reformulation throughout the school year, they have been unable to direct efforts to new product development to provide districts with additional food options that comply with the new requirements.

making them somewhat redundant.[14] Although this implies that USDA may permanently remove the meat and grain maximums, USDA officials told us that the Department is still considering options for a long-term solution to the meat and grain maximums and has not yet made a permanent decision.

None of the eight SFAs we visited made substantial changes to their menus in response to USDA's temporary removal of the weekly meat and grain maximums. Reasons that SFAs cited for this decision included: the flexibility was temporary, districts had already modified their menus to comply with the new requirements, products were already ordered for those menus, staff were already trained, and students had been educated about the new requirements. Instead, those SFAs that made some modifications after the flexibility was allowed focused on marginal changes that would ease menu planning and improve student acceptance of lunches. For example, in the district in which students reacted strongly to the decreased size of the tortilla wrap for sandwiches, the SFA brought in a larger wrap, though it was still smaller than the wrap used previously. Further, in the district that experienced a student boycott of lunch in part because of the change to the sub roll, the sub roll used in prior school years returned to the high school lunch menus. In another district that had decreased the amount of mini corn dogs they provided to each elementary school student because of the maximums, additional mini corn dogs were added to each student's portion.

SFA directors, food manufacturers, and other relevant industry representatives indicated the need for a timely and permanent federal decision on these maximums. Specifically, some SFA directors we visited told us that it is difficult to know how to proceed with menu planning under the new requirements when the flexibility provided over the maximums continues to be temporary. The School Nutrition Association, which represents SFAs across the country, has indicated that it supports the

---

[14] The Institute of Medicine report on which USDA based the new lunch requirements states that both the food component and calorie requirements are needed to achieve alignment with the Dietary Guidelines for Americans, which is why they recommended including both the calorie ranges and the weekly amounts for each food component, including meats and grains. However, although the Institute attempted to analyze the recommendations with respect to likely benefits and negative consequences, its report noted that the evidence on which to base such predictions is limited. As a result, the Institute may not have foreseen the operational challenges associated with the meat and grain maximums.

permanent elimination of the meat and grain maximums, because their removal will give cafeterias more flexibility to design healthy menus that meet nutrition standards and student tastes. Although the flexibility exists for school year 2013-2014, because USDA has given SFAs mixed messages regarding the Department's future plans for the meat and grain maximums, SFAs are currently left guessing about the future outcome, making planning future budgets and food ordering difficult. Several industry representatives said that because some SFAs are planning menus that comply with the maximums, while others are planning menus that include larger meat and grain portion sizes, industry is experiencing difficulties forecasting demand, which leads to food production, inventory, and storage challenges. This situation will soon become more complicated because of the impending federal changes to the content of meals served through the School Breakfast Program and other foods sold in schools.

Calorie Requirements for Middle and High Schools Also Challenged Some SFAs

Because the required calorie ranges for grades 6-8 and 9-12 do not overlap, schools with students in both these grade groups faced challenges complying with the calorie requirements. While the grades K-5 and 6-8 average daily calorie ranges for school lunches overlap at 550-650 and 600-700, the grades 6-8 and 9-12 ranges, which are 600-700 and 750-850, do not.[15] This creates a challenge for schools that include students from both grade groups, including schools in two of the districts we visited. One SFA director, whose district includes schools serving 7th through 12th graders, noted that complying with both of the calorie range requirements is particularly difficult when students in different grades use the same serving lines and share a lunch period. The director noted that cashiers at the point-of-sale may not know each student's grade level, which complicates the accurate identification of a meal that complies with the requirements. In addition, if certain food items are offered to some students and not to others depending on their grade, students may react negatively to the differential treatment. Because of these implementation issues, this district planned its menus to generally provide 725 calorie

[15] The Institute of Medicine report used data-based methods to provide a basis for the calculation of appropriate values for mean total daily calorie requirements for students in the three grade groups. Specifically, the report indicates that calorie range recommendations are based on reference growth chart data for healthy weights and heights, objective data on physical activity, and data on how calories are distributed among meals and snacks consumed by schoolchildren.

lunches for all students in these schools, which are not in compliance with either of the required ranges, and could potentially result in fiscal action against the SFA in the future.[16]

USDA's response to this issue, provided in part through the Department's guidance on menu planning under the new lunch requirements, has been limited. In the proposed rule on the new lunch requirements, USDA indicated that the new requirements are expected to bring about positive outcomes, including simplification of school lunch administration and operations. However, in comments on the proposed rule, some school districts expressed concerns that the lack of overlap in the calorie ranges may lead to increased costs and administrative burden. Although USDA did not change the ranges in the final rule, in its guidance on the new requirements, the Department acknowledges that the lack of overlap in the calorie ranges for these grade groups can be challenging. Because of this, USDA's guidance suggests that districts serve a menu appropriate for the lower grade level and add a few additional foods for students in the upper grade level. This differs from the previous requirements, which allowed schools to comply with meal requirements for the predominant grade group in schools that included students from two different groups. USDA's guidance also differs to some extent from the approach recommended by the Institute of Medicine in its report on which the federal requirements are based. The report's authors suggested that, for schools serving students from multiple grade groups on the same serving line, the SFA should work with the state agency to find a solution that ensures the basic elements of the standards for menu planning will be maintained, including moderate calorie values.

Student Acceptance Has Been a Challenge to Some Extent

While all eight SFAs we visited expressed support for the goal of improving the nutritional quality of lunches and felt the new requirements were moving in that direction, all eight experienced various challenges related to student acceptance of some of the foods served to comply with the requirements. Under the new requirements, lunches must include

---

[16] Under USDA regulations, an SFA found to have served meals not in compliance with requirements is potentially subject to fiscal action, such as the recovery of federal reimbursements for those meals.

whole grain-rich products and vegetables from 5 sub-groups each week,[17] and districts we visited noted that obtaining student acceptance of some whole grain-rich products and vegetables in the beans and peas (legumes) and red-orange sub-groups have been challenging. For example, six districts mentioned student acceptance of whole grain breads or pasta as being a challenge. Regarding vegetable sub-groups, five districts we visited said that they have had difficulty obtaining student acceptance of the beans and peas (legumes) sub-group, and two districts expressed difficulty with sweet potatoes, in the red-orange sub-group. Some noted that they have continued to try new recipes throughout the year to address these challenges, but acceptance has been limited. Challenges with student acceptance of these foods were foreseen by the Institute of Medicine in its report recommending they be required components of school lunch, as national data showed that few students reported eating these types of foods. The researchers noted that implementation of effective educational, marketing, and food preparation strategies, as well as the increased availability of suitable and appetizing products, may improve student acceptance of these foods.

Some districts reported that, if the past is an indicator, student acceptance of these foods may improve over time, and student comments regarding other healthy foods they like suggest this as well. In four of the districts we visited, SFA directors noted that they had begun adding whole grains into their menus before the current school year, and they have seen student acceptance of whole grain products improve over time. In addition, one district's SFA director also noted that acceptance of foods in the beans and peas (legumes) sub-group has improved over time. When we talked to students in the schools we visited and asked them about lunch foods they do not like, these specific foods were mentioned by some students in four of the eight districts, but most students focused their comments on other vegetables or specific entrees. Further, most of the students we talked to indicated that they like to eat healthy and nutritious foods, and they think that school lunches generally

---

[17] Regarding the grains component of the lunch, federal regulations require that all grain products must be made with enriched and whole grain meal or flour, and whole grain-rich products must contain at least 51 percent whole grains. Beginning July 1, 2012, half of the grain products offered during the school week must meet the whole grain-rich criteria, and beginning July 1, 2014, all grain products must meet these criteria. Regarding the vegetables component of the lunch, federal regulations define the minimum weekly serving sizes for each of the vegetable sub-groups—dark green vegetables, red-orange vegetables, beans and peas (legumes), starchy vegetables, and other vegetables.

provide such foods. Although school year 2012-2013 is the first year that students were required to take a fruit or a vegetable with school lunch nationwide, when we asked students what they like about school lunch this year, students in 13 of the 17 schools we visited to observe lunch reported liking certain fruit and vegetable options.

Food waste is also an indicator of lack of student acceptance of the new lunch requirements. Students may take the food components they are required to as part of the school lunch, but they may then choose not to consume them. Although none of the districts we visited had fully analyzed food waste over the past few years to determine if it changed during school year 2012-2013,[18] six of the SFAs we visited told us they believe food waste has increased because of the new lunch requirements. In particular, SFAs said that the fruits and vegetables students are now required to take sometimes end up thrown away, and in our lunch period observations in 7 of 17 schools, we saw many students throw some or all of their fruits and vegetables away. However, at the same time, we observed other students take and consume sizable quantities of fruits and vegetables and the other lunch components in the remaining 10 schools in which we observed lunch, resulting in minimal food waste. Four of the SFAs we visited talked about food waste being more of an issue with the youngest elementary school students, possibly because of the amount of food served with the lunch and the amount of time they have to consume it. The Institute of Medicine report acknowledged differences in food intake among elementary students, noting that the amounts of food offered under the new recommendations may be too large for some of the younger elementary school children because they are more likely to have lower energy needs than the older children in the same grade group. In USDA's final rule, the Department discussed the offer versus serve policy, which has been required for senior high schools and optional for all other schools since 1975, as a way to minimize food waste. Under the current regulations, this policy allows students to decline two of the five meal components offered with the lunch, rather than requiring students to be served all five components.[19] However, the SFA director in one of the districts we visited

---

[18] One of the districts we visited has been working with a university researcher on a plate waste study, but a final report has yet to be issued.

[19] However, under the current regulations, students must select at least ½ cup of the fruit or vegetable component with their lunches.

noted that the district has chosen not to implement the offer versus serve policy for the youngest students because they have difficulty making choices, which extends the time spent in the serving line and decreases the time students have to consume their lunch.

Student participation in lunch has decreased to some extent in school year 2012-2013, which is another indicator that student acceptance of school lunches may have declined since the changes. Most of the SFAs we visited reported that they experienced decreases in lunch participation in school year 2012-2013 in part because of the new lunch requirements and other factors.[20] USDA's national data, which do not account for adjustments related to changes in monthly serving days or student enrollment across years, also generally show that student lunch participation was lower in school year 2012-2013 than it was the year before. Later this year, when we complete our study of the school lunch changes, we plan to provide additional information on lunch participation trends.

SFAs Faced Other Challenges, Including Hunger Concerns and Increased Costs

SFAs also faced concerns in school year 2012-2013 that the new lunch requirements were leaving some students hungry—an issue raised in five of the districts we visited. For example, in one district, a high school principal told us that during school year 2012-2013, athletic coaches expressed concerns that student athletes were hungrier after school than they were in previous years, and staff reported that more students were distracted during the final period of the school day than in previous years. In the district we visited in which middle and high school students boycotted school lunch at the beginning of the year, the boycott was led by two student athletes in part because they indicated that the lunches were leaving them hungry. These concerns were likely related to decreased entrée sizes. During our visits to schools, students in six schools mentioned that they have been hungry this year after eating school lunch because of various reasons. For example, students in three schools attributed this to the smaller entrees, and students in one of those schools also noted that it may be related to the timing of their lunch periods, as their school's first lunch period began around 10:30 a.m. and the school day ended at about 2:30 p.m. In another school, students

---

[20] While we obtained some lunch participation data from the districts we visited, we have not yet fully analyzed the changes they experienced.

acknowledged that they had not taken or eaten all of the items offered with the lunch, which we observed resulted in a smaller sized lunch. (See figure 1.) In contrast, when students served themselves all of the lunch components in the districts that we visited, their lunches were substantially larger in size, primarily because of the large amounts of fruits and vegetables they selected. (See figure 2.)

Figure 1: Three Food Component Lunches

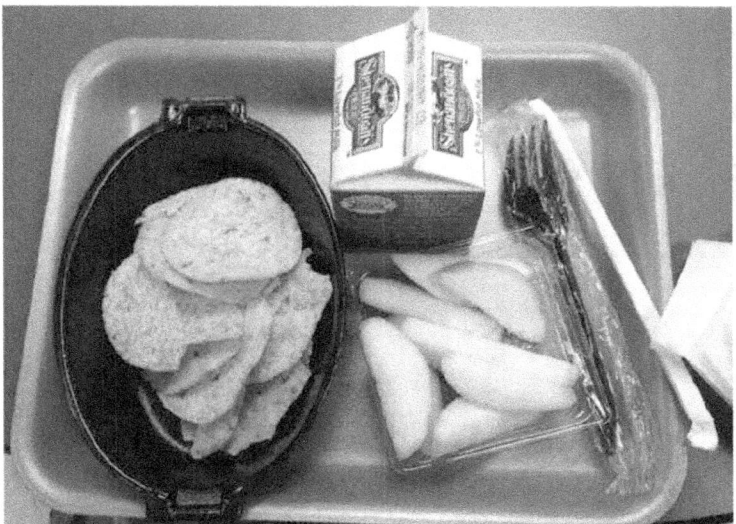 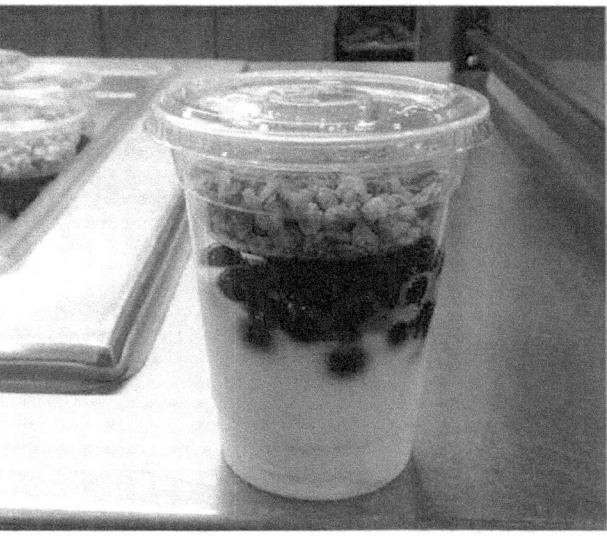

Source: GAO.

Note: Food components included in the lunches shown are: grain, fruit, and milk in the lunch on the left; and grain, fruit, and meat alternate (yogurt) in the lunch on the right.

Figure 2: Five Food Component Lunches

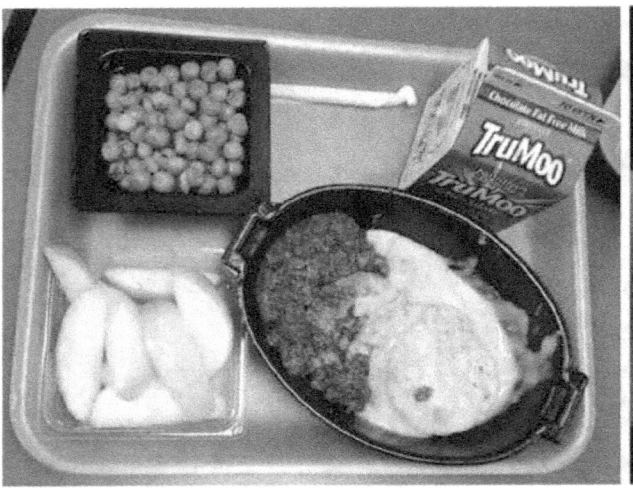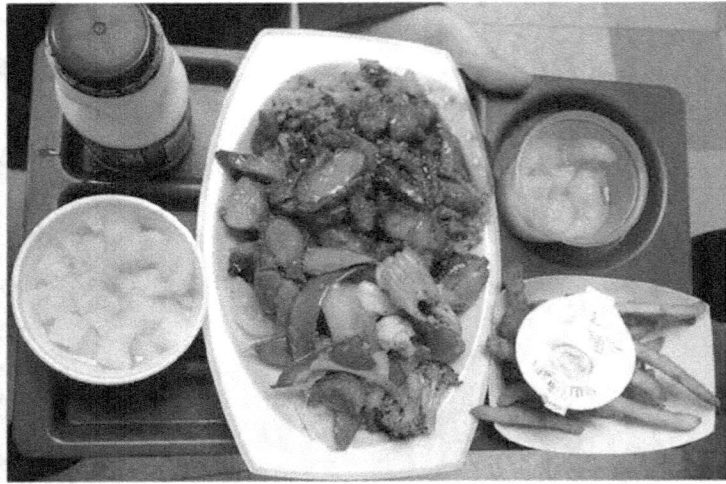

Source: GAO.

Note: Food components included in both the lunches shown are grain, meat/meat alternate, fruit, vegetable, and mi k.

School lunches generally provide fewer calories under the new requirements than in past years, likely because of smaller entrée sizes. Specifically, the new required lunch calorie maximums for each grade group are either lower or comparable to the calorie minimums previously required. As a result, school lunches generally provided more calories in the past, according to national data, than they are allowed to in school year 2012-2013, particularly for younger students.[21] Although the previous nutrition standards were developed to align school lunches with the Dietary Guidelines for Americans, they were developed in the mid 1990s. Since then, the percentage of children who are overweight and obese has increased, and research has shown that excess food consumption, poor food choices, and decreased physical activity contribute to these trends. The Institute of Medicine's 2010 recommendations for the lunch pattern were developed using a data-

---

[21] National data from school year 2009-2010 show that the average calorie content of school lunch offered was 726 in elementary schools, 785 in middle schools, and 843 in high schools; see *School Nutrition Dietary Assessment Study IV, 2012.* The average daily maximum calorie content for lunches under the new federal requirements is: 650 for grades K-5, 700 for grades 6-8 and 850 for grades 9-12.

based approach, which assessed data on healthy weights and heights, physical activity, and the distribution of calories among meals, and the authors indicate that the recommended lunches are appropriate for the level of physical activity of most children.

SFAs also expressed concerns about the impact of compliance with the new lunch requirements on food costs and their budgets. All eight SFAs we visited reported that they have incurred increases in fruit and vegetable costs this year because of the requirement that students take at least one fruit or vegetable with lunch. Further, most indicated that overall costs for school lunch were greater in school year 2012-2013 than in the past, and three expressed concerns about the impact of these changes on their overall financial stability. Because we conducted our visits before the end of the school year, we have not yet obtained data from these SFAs on how they ended the year financially, though we plan to provide information on those results in our final report.

All eight SFAs we visited also discussed other challenges implementing the lunch changes during school year 2012-2013, such as additional menu planning issues, food procurement, new requirements related to the price of lunches, the pace of implementation, and USDA's assistance with the changes. When we complete our study of the lunch changes later this year, we will provide additional information about implementation challenges and USDA's assistance to states and SFAs with implementation.

SFAs Noted Concerns about the Proposed Competitive Foods Changes

In addition to the school lunch changes, the Healthy Hunger-Free Kids Act of 2010 required that USDA specify and require nutrition standards for all foods and beverages sold outside the school meals programs on the school campus during the school day, which are commonly referred to as competitive foods because they compete with school meal programs. Competitive foods are often sold through vending machines, school stores, and fundraisers, and also include SFA sales of a la carte items in the cafeteria. In school year 2009-2010, competitive foods were sold in an estimated 93 percent of schools nationwide, according to a recent USDA study.[22] The proposed rule containing these standards was published by

---

[22] *School Nutrition Dietary Assessment Study IV (2012).*

USDA in February 2013,[23] and during our visits to SFAs, many expressed concerns that certain aspects of the proposed rule would be challenging to implement, if finalized.[24]

Specifically, seven of the eight SFAs we visited expressed concerns about what they viewed as a lack of clarity in the proposed rule regarding how the nutrition standards for competitive food sales administered by entities other than the SFA will be enforced. In our 2005 report on competitive foods,[25] we found that many different people made decisions about competitive food sales, but no one person commonly had responsibility for all sales in a school. At that time, in a majority of schools nationwide, district officials made competitive food policies, while SFA directors and principals made decisions about specific sales. Other groups, such as student clubs and booster groups, also made competitive food decisions through their direct involvement in sales. The number and variety of groups involved in these sales typically increased as the school level increased. For example, an estimated 48 percent of middle schools nationwide had three or more groups involved in these sales compared to an estimated 83 percent of high schools. Although a 2004 law required districts to implement wellness policies in school year 2006-2007 that addressed nutritional guidelines for all foods available in schools during the school day, some of the SFAs we recently visited told us that these policies have generally not been enforced, in part because no one person was granted enforcement responsibility over all such sales.[26]

---

[23] National School Lunch Program and School Breakfast Program: Nutrition Standards for All Foods Sold In School as Required by the Healthy, Hunger-Free Kids Act of 2010, 78 Fed. Reg. 9530 (proposed Feb. 8, 2013) (to be codified at 7 C.F.R. pts. 210 and 220).

[24] USDA sought public comments on the proposed rule and will consider these comments in finalizing the rule. For purposes of this testimony, we did not review or analyze the comments submitted in response to the proposed rulemaking. To view the comments that were submitted in response to the proposed rule, visit www.regulations.gov. The comments described in this testimony were shared with us by SFAs during our site visits and may or may not echo themes that were raised by those officially commenting on the proposed rule.

[25] GAO, School Meal Programs: Competitive Foods are Widely Available and Generate Substantial Revenues for Schools, GAO-05-563 (Washington, D.C.: Aug. 8, 2005).

[26] Recognizing this, as part of a broader city campaign on health and wellness, one of the districts we visited recently created a separate department responsible for health and wellness initiatives, including enforcement of the district's wellness policy and nutritional guidelines for all foods sold in schools.

SFAs we visited also expressed concern that the proposed rule's inclusion of differing nutrition standards based on the type of competitive foods sale will put the SFA at a competitive disadvantage relative to other food sales within a school. For example, five SFA directors expressed concerns about the proposed rule's provision allowing states discretion to make decisions about fundraisers that are exempt from the federal nutrition standards for competitive foods. Some SFA directors expressed concerns that this would potentially result in inconsistent treatment, whereby SFAs' competitive food sales would be required to follow the nutrition standards and fundraisers would not. Similarly, some SFAs expressed concerns about the proposed rule's inclusion of different standards for beverages sold in food service areas during meal periods—which are typically sold through SFA a la carte sales—and beverages sold outside of meal service areas—such as those through vending machines. Specifically, although the proposed rule allows the sale of milk, water, and juice through any competitive food venue at any time, the rule also allows the sale of other beverages, except for in food service areas during meal periods. However, this restriction is somewhat similar to the current federal requirements on competitive food sales.[27]

Conclusions

Across the country, more nutritious school lunches likely were provided to students during school year 2012-2013. All eight SFAs we visited expressed support for the goal of improving the nutritional quality of lunches and felt the new federal requirements were moving in that direction. Many students' positive comments on healthy foods, their views that school lunches generally provide such foods, and their consumption of sizeable quantities of fruits and vegetables in the majority of schools we visited indicate that acceptance of the new lunch requirements will improve over time. However, as the first year of implementation of the new requirements for the content of school lunches has unfolded, the SFAs we visited also faced a variety of challenges.

While some of the challenges SFAs faced this year have been addressed and others may become less difficult as time elapses, those caused by the required weekly maximum amounts of meats and grains permitted in lunches and the lack of overlap in the allowable calorie ranges for grades

---

[27] Currently, federal regulations prohibit the sale of certain competitive foods, known as foods of minimal nutritional value (FMNV), during meal periods in school cafeterias and other food service areas. FMNV, as defined by USDA, include soda, chewing gum, and hard candy, for example.

6-8 and 9-12 likely will not. Because of the meat and grain maximums, some districts made menu decisions that are inconsistent with the goal of improving children's diets, as they added desserts and condiments that increased the amount of sugar, salt, or fat in lunches in order to comply with the required calorie minimums. Acknowledging that the meat and grain maximums created challenges for SFAs, USDA lifted them through school year 2013-2014 and indicated that the maximums may not be needed to accomplish the nutrition goals of the new requirements. However, although USDA has acknowledged the need for a permanent decision on the maximums, they have yet to provide one, hindering the ability of school districts to plan menus, food purchases, budgets, staff training, and student education because they do not know whether the meat and grain restrictions will be reinstated in the future or not. In addition, the requirements that lunches served to students in grades 6-8 provide different amounts of calories than lunches served to students in grades 9-12—even in schools that serve students in both grade groups—is inconsistent with past practices, expert recommendations, and USDA's intent of simplifying the administration and operations of the school lunch program. Most significantly, the inflexibility of these calorie requirements substantially hinders certain SFAs' ability to comply, which may potentially result in fiscal action against SFAs in future years. Absent a permanent USDA decision to remove the meat and grain maximums and increase flexibility for schools that serve meals to students in both the 6-8 and 9-12 grade groupings, SFAs will continue to face challenges implementing the regulations, potentially impeding their efforts to meet their key goals—healthier foods in school for healthier students.

Recommendations

To improve SFAs' ability to design menus that comply with the new lunch requirements, we recommend that the Secretary of Agriculture:

- permanently remove the weekly meat/meat alternate and grain maximums for school lunch defined in federal regulations, and
- modify federal regulations or guidance to allow school districts flexibility in complying with the defined calorie ranges for schools with students in both the grades 6-8 and 9-12 groups.

We provided a draft of this testimony to USDA for review and comment. In oral comments, USDA officials indicated that they generally agreed with our recommendation regarding meats and grains, and they are currently developing an approach for permanently lifting the meat and grain maximums. Officials added that while they recognize the need to address the challenges posed by lack of overlap in the calorie ranges for grades 6-8 and 9-12, it is important to identify a solution to this issue that ensures calorie ranges remain appropriately targeted to students based on their ages—a point emphasized by the Institute of Medicine. USDA officials also said that they have been collecting information on implementation of the new lunch requirements throughout the year from many school districts and have heard about implementation challenges. However, according to USDA officials, official reporting by states indicates that a majority of districts have been able to comply with the new requirements. USDA also expressed concern that the findings in the testimony did not reflect a nationally representative sample of school districts. We continue to believe that our site visits to eight school districts and our interviews with eight SFA directors from across the country, state officials, and industry representatives enabled us to identify some of the challenges school districts are facing in implementing the new nutrition standards. Our final report will provide additional information and data to inform these issues.

Chairman Rokita and Members of the Subcommittee, this concludes my statement. I would be pleased to respond to questions you may have.

Contacts and Staff Acknowledgments

For further questions on this testimony, please contact me at (202) 512-7215 or brownke@gao.gov. Contact points for our Offices of Congressional Relations and Public Affairs may be found on the last page of this statement. Individuals who made key contributions to this statement include Jessica Botsford, Robert Campbell, Rachel Frisk, Kathy Larin, Jean McSween, Dan Meyer, and Zachary Sivo.